DR BARBARA LYME DISEASE DIET FOR BEGINNERS

A Simple Guide To Repair Lyme Disease Through Dr Barbara Alkaline Plant-Based Diet Without Negative Effects

KATHONA BODI

ISBN: 9798333380661

CONTENTS

Introduction 7

Let's Start With the Basics 10

What Is The Lyme Diet? 14

Using the Dr Barbara Diet for Lyme Disease 20

Additional Tips for Fighting Lyme Disease 27

Dr Barbara Alkaline Recipes for Lyme Disease 31

Conclusion 71

Introduction

Recently, there seems to be an upsurge in Lyme disease cases and other tick-borne related conditions. In fact, in the US alone, reports show that about three hundred thousand cases are recorded yearly.

In reality, the number may be actually more than that. You may not believe it but over 1.5 million people are dealing with Lyme disease. This should explain why many and more people are educating themselves about the illness.

If you are part of this statistics or know someone living with the disease, you might be wondering if making changes to your diet can have any impact on your recovery. Well, it's no news that people with certain illnesses often have to switch to a specific diet in an attempt to manage the condition or support their recovery. This is no different with Lyme disease.

Lyme disease is linked to chronic inflammation. When you're in this state, the last thing you want to do is make poor dietary choices as this is like fueling a burning fire. It will only get worse!

The good news is that following a proper diet can help ease the symptoms of Lyme disease and support your healing process while improving your overall health. That is the whole idea behind Dr Barbara's Alkaline Diet Guide.

Let's Start With the Basics

Let's start by answering an important question. What is Lyme disease?

Like most health problems, Lyme disease is directly linked to chronic inflammation. It is an infection brought about by a bacterium known as Borrelia burgdorferi. It is typically contracted when you're bitten by a tick carrying this bacteria, which in most cases are deer ticks (also known as black-legged ticks).

When this happens, the bacteria is transmitted into the bloodstream and then immediately begin to multiply and fill up locations where they may not be detected by antibiotics.

Interestingly, when your body becomes aware of such a threat, it immediately switches into a protective mode and produces inflammation.

This inflammation, which is the body's natural response to infection, illness, or injury, tries to hunt down the bacteria and get rid of it. Unfortunately, the bacteria may take cover in the scar tissue around the joints, where they are protected by biofilms. This can make them undiscoverable by inflammation.

The problem is that inflammation usually doesn't give up. It will continue to look for these bacteria and will only stop when it feels the problem has been taken care of. The implication is that your body will continue to get inflamed.

The good news is that there are certain things you can do to reduce this inflammation, and it all starts with changing your diet.

How to Know You Have Lyme Disease

So, what are the symptoms of Lyme disease?

The more common symptom of Lyme disease when in development is usually a rash which typically occurs around the original area of the tick bite, but this may not always be the case.

Besides a rash, there are several other symptoms associated with the disease depending on what stage it is.

Here are the more common ones:

- Stiffness of the neck
- Headache (usually very severe)
- Brain fog
- Autoimmunity
- Chronic fatigue
- Fever
- Depression & Anxiety
- Feeling dizzy most of the time
- Joint pain or arthritis (which may come with swelling)
- Nerve damage
- Shortness of breath
- Arrhythmia
- The brain or spinal cord can become inflamed

As you can see, these symptoms can affect one's quality of life and can be difficult to manage.

Most people explore various treatment options in an attempt to recover or at least experience some relief. One of these treatments is nutrition!

What Is The Lyme Diet?

People who have Lyme disease usually have their immune system greatly impacted. As a result, it's important you do everything possible to support the immune systems, as this will prove beneficial in managing the symptoms.

Another thing you may want to consider is inflammation. As earlier indicated, chronic inflammation is usually the chief cause of Lyme disease, so it only makes sense to consider an anti-inflammatory diet when seeking to reduce the symptoms.

In general, most Lyme disease sufferers often opt for antibiotic treatment but this is hardly enough to address the problem in most cases.

Tenets of the Lyme Diet

While everyone's needs might not exactly be the same, a Lyme diet should have these basic tenets:

Must support the immune system

When you have Lyme disease, it is very important you avoid foods that suppress the immune system. As you already know, the number one food in this category is sugar.

You must limit your intake of refined sugar or completely cut it off from your diet. Besides weakening the immune system, sugar can also feed candida.

Not only refined sugar but also alcohol, beverages, and processed foods. All these can feed candida which can worsen inflammation.

Specifically, sugar tends to feed the biofilms protecting the bacteria, which makes it harder for them to be broken down by antibiotics or other medications.

With this in mind, it is better to avoid sugar when you have Lyme disease. Even natural sugar from fruits can be a problem, especially if you're taking antibiotics and have a candida problem.

So, even though the Dr Barbara diet incorporates alkaline fruits, I highly recommend you reduce your fruit intake. Ideally, you should opt for lesser-sweet fruits.

Besides exacerbating inflammation, other effects of consuming sugary foods and drinks include:

- Dysregulation of hormones
- Creating spikes in your blood sugar levels
- And several other health problems

In fact, the effect of sugar can be worse if you already have an existing condition in addition to Lyme disease.

You may not know this, but sugar can trigger the release of free fatty acids in the liver, which also encourages inflammation.

Must contain little to no gluten

Gluten is another "monster" you must avoid when you have Lyme disease. This is because, like sugar, gluten can increase the amount of inflammation in the body.

Many people do not even know that they are gluten-intolerant, and this is because it doesn't always come with digestive symptoms.

In general, you want to reduce your gluten intake. This includes things like rye, barley, bread, crackers, cookies, wheat, oats, and other carb-filled foods or those made from flour.

While these foods taste nice, they are not always good for the body.

Like sugar, gluten can activate the immune system, which creates a big problem when you're dealing with Lyme disease.

Besides its impact on Lyme disease sufferers, excess gluten can also contribute to other illnesses such as ulcerative colitis, psoriasis, thyroid disorder, celiac disease, multiple sclerosis, and so on.

The last thing you want is to be dealing with any of these while also having Lyme disease.

The Dr Barbara diet guide mainly focuses on consuming plant-based foods.

However, if you're heavily invested in processed foods, then you should start examining labels to identify where the gluten is. These include food and beverages, and even toiletries.

Well, if you're reading this book, I'm guessing you've made up your mind to do plants. If that is the case, then we have no business talking about processed foods.

No dairy

For most Lyme disease patients, the general recommendation will usually be to reduce dairy.

But if you're serious about following Dr Barbara's recommendations, then you should consider cutting it out from your diet completely. Yes, eliminate dairy from your diet.

The main reason why you should avoid dairy is because, like sugar and gluten, it is inflammatory. And for someone with Lyme disease, you want to avoid anything that can exacerbate your inflammation.

Using the Dr Barbara Diet for Lyme Disease

Like I said earlier, when you have a problem with inflammation, the last thing you want to do is feed poorly. Doing so will be like pouring fuel on an already burning fire. So, what do you do instead?

Well, you simply switch to a proper diet, ideally one that is proven to reduce chronic inflammation. I'm talking about the Dr Barbara diet.

Who Is Dr Barbara?

Well, as you would expect, Dr Barbara O'Neill is the brain behind the Dr Barbara Diet. She's an advocate for alternatives and a well-known nutritionist who believes in the power of food to heal diseases.

Dr Barbara has over four decades of experience in the health industry, which makes her teachings valuable as she has helped a lot of people achieve optimal health naturally without the use of drugs.

So, *what is the Dr Barbara Diet?*

The Dr. Barbara diet is essentially a plant-based way of eating that focuses on consuming high-fiber, alkaline-rich foods from plant-based sources, and minimal processed foods. The diet typically consists of legumes, whole grains, fruits, vegetables, as well as nuts and seeds.

According to Barbara, eating this way helps to balance and maintain the body's pH levels, which promotes optimal health and helps to prevent or heal from diseases.

Why Does the Dr Barbara Diet Work for Lyme Disease?

One of the reasons why the Dr Barbara diet works so well for Lyme disease is because it's rich in fiber.

Fiber-rich foods are required to keep the intestinal tract healthy. You may be wondering - how is this connected to Lyme disease?

Well, to heal from Lyme disease, you need healthy digestion and good bowel function. In fact, this doesn't only apply to Lyme disease but any other illness.

Another reason the Dr Barbara diet plan works so well is because it's anti-inflammatory.

Since Lyme disease is associated with chronic inflammation, you need a diet that can help reduce the inflammation rather than exacerbate it.

The Dr Barbara diet is also nutrient-dense, which makes it a good maintenance diet for your general health and well-being.

Some examples of nutrient-dense, anti-inflammatory foods include:

- Berries

- Legumes
- Foods rich in health fats and Omega-3 such as flaxseed and flax oil, olive oil, and avocado
- Fresh vegetables and leafy greens

Furthermore, in addition to "sweeping" the intestines, some fiber can also nourish good bacteria, which promotes a healthy microbiome.

In turn, this strengthens the mucosal barrier and helps in preventing a leaky gut; all of which are required to maintain a strong immune system.

Some Special Vitamin-Rich Foods for Lyme Disease

Some foods contain some macronutrients that may be beneficial to Lyme disease sufferers. Some of them are listed below:

Vitamin D rich foods such as:

- Mushroom
- Plant milk

- Fortified breakfast cereal
- Spinach
- Amaranth
- Chia seeds
- Fortified orange juice
- Etc.

Vitamin A rich foods such as:

- Sweet potatoes
- Mango
- Papaya
- Squash
- Guava
- Kale
- Spinach
- Carrots
- Cantaloupe
- Red pepper
- Pumpkin
- Lettuce
- Etc.

Vitamin C rich foods such as:

- Peppers

- Brussel sprouts

- Citrus fruits

- Broccoli

- Strawberries

- Kale

- Cabbage

- Kiwi

- Tomatoes

- Cauliflower

- Pineapple

- Raspberries

- Watercress

- Etc.

Glutamine-rich foods such as:

- Nuts (such as almonds and cashews)

- Seeds (such as sunflower seeds and pumpkin seeds)

- Banana

- Onions

* Red cabbage
* Legumes such as peas, lentils and chickpeas
* Parsley
* Etc.

Selenium-rich foods such as:

* Brazil nuts
* Cereals and other whole grains
* Brown rice
* Fresh bananas
* Barley
* Pasta
* Sesame seeds
* Sunflower seeds
* Mushrooms
* Etc.

Additional Tips for Fighting Lyme Disease

In addition to a healthy diet, there are other things you could do to help your Lyme treatment. Let's briefly look at them:

Reduce stress

As with many other illnesses, stress is a big issue when it comes to Lyme disease. This is because the infection usually creates stress and some treatments may be lengthy, which can cause additional stress.

Even as you've decided to follow a plant-based diet, it's important to realize that it might take some time to see results.

So, it's important you develop a coping mechanism and reduce other sources of stress in your life, especially in your day-to-day activities.

Drink enough water

Staying hydrated is very important when you're dealing with Lyme as water is another great way to reduce inflammation.

As earlier indicated, avoid unhealthy drinks such as coffee, canned juices, soda, and other sugary drinks. Instead, opt for natural juices and smoothies from fresh fruits and vegetables. I have included a lot of recipes to help you get started.

In general, it's best you make your own drinks from fresh fruits and vegetables.

Start with the basics

Before you start following the Dr Barbara diet, it's important you start with the foundation foods.

Specifically, you want to cut out foods or substances that can potentially trigger inflammation and weaken your immune system. Sugar is usually the number one culprit.

Other foods you should avoid include saturated fats, foods that are hard to digest or make you feel bad after eating them, packaged foods, processed foods, etc.

Also, you may need to avoid food that could be potential allergens such as eggs, fish, tree nuts, corn, wheat/gluten, etc.

Combine your diet with fasting

When it comes to general wellness, fasting can be a game-changer. In fact, apart from fighting off disease, fasting is a great way to maintain the immune system.

Observing regular periods of fasting, especially at the initial stages of Lyme can fasten your recovery.

There are different types of fasting - dry fasting, water fasting, and intermittent fasting.

Any of these is acceptable depending on your schedule, however, I have found that a 24-hour dry fast two or three times a week is a great way to go. If you don't think you can go that long without food, then you can try intermittent fasting. You can find out more about the different types of fast. I have a whole chapter on fasting in some of my other books.

In general, whether you're fasting or not, if you're following the Dr Barbara diet, you are expected to eat only two normal meals and one light meal a day.

Personally, I would recommend not eating more than two normal meals daily. During my own health battles, I would eat just once (or none) and fast the rest of the day. When you are starting out, you want to spend more time fasting.

Dr Barbara Alkaline Recipes for Lyme Disease

GRANOLA PLATE

Things You Need

- Two and a half cups of oats
- A cup of shredded coconut, unsweetened without preservatives
- 1 tsp of vanilla, extract
- ¾ cup of almonds
- ¼ cup of maple syrup (should be pure)
- ¼ cup of pumpkin seeds
- ½ cup of walnuts (only use if you tolerate it)
- ¼ tsp cinnamon (optional)
- ⅛ tsp of sea salt
- 2 tbsp of coconut oil
- Dried mango to taste (optional, must come without any preservatives)

Cooking Instructions

1. Start by preheating your oven. Set the temperature at 300 degrees Fahrenheit.
2. Transfer the almonds, oats, and walnuts onto cookie sheet.
3. Next, get a small pot and mix the other ingredients - coconut oil, syrup, cinnamon, salt and vanilla. Now pour the mixture on top of the oats and walnuts and flip to mix it up.
4. Then bake for 18-22 minutes. Make sure to stir every 8-10 minutes.
5. When you're done, take it out of the oven, then add the pumpkin seeds and coconut.
6. Bake for an extra 10 to 15 minutes, then take it out and move to a Pyrex dish to get it to cool. Once again, you want to stir often.
7. Optionally, you can cut the dried mango into tiny slices and mix with the granola. Otherwise, skip this step if it's not tolerated. Put it in the fridge to cool.

"MINT" ICED TEA

Things You Need

- 1 tbsp of mint leaves (fresh, ideally should come in a sachet or tea ball)
- Chamomile tea (a bag should be enough)
- 1 teaspoon of sweetener (agave syrup/you can also use raw honey though this is not permitted in Dr Sebi's guide)

Cooking Instructions

1. Get a medium-sized teapot and fill it with water. Now, soak (or steep) the tea for 18-20 minutes.
2. Remove the mint and chamomile. Add your preferred sweetener and stir well. Allow it to cool down, then put it in the fridge.

WATERMELON SALAD

Things You Need

- One red watermelon (small or half-size, seedless)
- One to two cups of English cucumber (sliced)
- Mint sprigs to taste (make sure it's fresh)
- ***Blueberries (one half-pint box)***

Cooking Instructions

1. Slice the watermelon into tiny pieces. Next, "scrape off" the outer part, then cut into very small chunks.
2. Transfer the chunks to 1 large bowl or you can divide it into smaller bowls.
3. Next, add the cucumber slices and use the blueberries and sprigs as toppings.

AVOCADO BOWL

Ingredients

- Fresh lime juice from 1 lime
- ½ cup cucumber, chopped
- 2 tbsp melted coconut oil
- 16-20 basil leaves (can be substituted with parsley leaves)
- 1 avocado
- Nuts, chopped
- ⅛ tsp lime zest (you can use more for serving)
- 1 pinch salt
- Agave to taste (optional)

Instructions

1. Start by pouring the lime juice into a blender. Add the avocado and agave. Then blend the mixture until smooth.
2. Now, add the lime zest, cucumber, salt, and coconut oil. Blend again until smooth.
3. Then add the basil or parsley leaves and mix a bit.
4. Transfer to a bowl and top with the chopped nuts. You can top with more lime zest if desired.

FRUIT SALAD

Ingredients

- One pint of fresh blueberries

- One ripe pear, cored and diced

- One pint of fresh strawberries, sliced (no stems)

- Two cups grapes, deseeded

- 2 tbsp date syrup (optional)

- ¼ tsp ground cinnamon

- 2 tbsp freshly squeezed lemon juice

Instructions

1. Combine all the ingredients in a bowl. Store in a refrigerator. Serve chill.

HERBERT HUMMUS

Ingredients

- Two garlic cloves
- One cup of fresh basil leaves, blanched and lightly packed
- Four cups of cooked garbanzo beans
- Juice from one lemon
- One cup of vegetable broth
- Half a cup of tarragon leaves, blanched and lightly packed
- Half a cup of fresh, flat parsley leaves
- ¼ cup of chives, chopped
- 2 tbsp sesame seeds, toasted

Instructions

1. Start by dabbing the basil leaves and tarragon until they dry. Now, cut them into smaller bits and put in a blender or food processor.

2. Add in the beans, sesame seeds, lemon juice, garlic, and vegetable broth. Blend until smooth and creamy. Add the chives; stir and serve.

NB: Consume within 4 days.

MISO NOODLE SOUP

Ingredients

- Two scallions, sliced
- One cup of adzuki beans (cooked or canned)
- Four tablespoons of miso
- Two tablespoons of fresh cilantro/basil, chopped
- Seven ounces of soba noodles (100% buckwheat)
- Four cups of water

Instructions

1. Start by pouring some water into a large pot; bring it to a boil.

2. Next, add in the soba noodles and stir. Cook for about five minutes, then drain and rinse (use hot water).

3. In another pot, pour in some water and bring to boil. Remove from heat and add in the miso and stir until dissolved.

4. Finally, add the noodles, adzuki beans, scallions and cilantro to the miso broth. Stir well to combine. Serve warm.

HEMP MILK

Ingredients

- Spring water
- 6 tbsp sea moss gel
- 1 cup hemp seeds

Instructions

1. Start by soaking the hemp seeds in 6 cups of spring water for 30 minutes.
2. Next, transfer the seeds with the water into a blender and blend until smooth.
3. Add in the sea moss and blend for 30 seconds. Store in the refrigerator and use within four days.

LEMON BRUSSEL SPROUTS

Ingredients

- ¼ cup fresh lemon juice
- Half a cup of chicken broth or low-sodium vegetable broth
- Zest from one lemon

- Two pounds of Brussel sprouts, the ends should be trimmed
- Two teaspoons of kosher salt
- ¼ teaspoon of fresh ground pepper

Instructions

1. Start by shredding the sprouts; you can do this with the slicing disk on a food processor or a sharp knife. If you're using a sharp knife, you will need to halve the sprouts before thinly slicing by hand.
2. Pour the broth into a deep skillet and heat over medium heat. Once it begins to simmer, add in the shredded sprouts and season with the pepper and salt.
3. Sauté and stir frequently until the sprouts become a little wilted. This should take about 8-10 minutes. Then remove the skillet from heat.
4. You can stir in the lemon zest and juice if you plan to serve right away, otherwise stir in the lemon just before you serve it hot or warm anytime.

PECANS & BERRIES SALAD

Ingredients

- Baby arugula or mixed baby greens (15 oz pack)

- Blackberries (half pack, should weigh up to 3 oz)

- Raspberries (half pack, should weigh up to 3 oz)

- Fifteen pecan halves

To make the vinaigrette, here's what you need:

- 3 tbsp extra virgin olive oil

- ⅛ tsp kosher salt

- ⅛ tsp freshly ground pepper to taste

- 1 tbsp champagne vinegar (or rice vinegar/ apple cider vinegar)

- ½ tsp dried basil

Instructions

1. Let's start with the dressing/vinaigrette. Pour the vinegar into a bowl (make sure it's a bowl that won't react with the vinegar). Now add in the basil, pepper, and salt.

2. Next, you want to emulsify the olive oil with the vinaigrette. To do this, drizzle the oil in a slow stream; then whisk together until emulsified.

3. Now, combine the vinaigrette and baby arugula (or mixed greens) and transfer to a salad bowl.

4. Top with pecans, raspberries, and blackberries. Serve immediately.

BUTTERNUT SQUASH SOUP

Ingredients

- One tablespoon of olive oil
- One small onion, chopped
- Two tablespoons of fresh sage, chopped

- Six cups of butternut squash (peeled and cubed, should weigh about 30 oz)
- Half a teaspoon of kosher salt or sea salt
- One sweet apple (ideally, it should be large in size, you will need to peel and chop it)
- Half a teaspoon of cinnamon, grounded
- Half a teaspoon of paprika
- Four and a half cups of vegetable broth
- One tablespoon of fresh ginger, grated
- Half a cup of coconut milk (you can use more for garnish)
- ¼ tsp fresh nutmeg, grated

Instructions

1. Start by preheating your oven to 400 degrees F. Next, mix the apple, sage, squash, cinnamon, onion, paprika, and ¼ tsp salt in a Dutch oven. Toss in one tablespoon of olive oil and combine very well.
2. Roast until the squash becomes tender. This usually takes about half an hour.

3. After that, transfer the Dutch oven to the stove and add in the coconut milk, broth, nutmeg, ginger, and ¼ tsp salt. Allow to boil.

4. Next, you want to blend the mixture. You can either use an immersion blender or you can transfer the soup to the blender in batches. Blend until you get a smooth consistency.

5. When serving, you can drizzle extra coconut milk on top and if you like, add a pinch of nutmeg.

CARROT BANANA PROTEIN DRINK

Ingredients

- ¼ cup unflavored pea protein powder (you can substitute this with whey protein)
- Half a teaspoon of turmeric
- One cup of almond milk

- One medium-sized banana, riped

- Two baby carrots

- One tablespoon of ground flax

- Agave syrup (or any other natural sweetener of your choice)

- Ice

Instructions

1. Add all the ingredients to a blender and blend until you get a smooth consistency. Enjoy!

SUPERFOOD SMOOTHIE

Ingredients

- 1 date, pitted

- Half medium-sized banana, riped

- Half a tablespoon of chia seeds

- One tablespoon of raw shelled hemp seeds (you can substitute this with any other seed of your choice)

- ¾ cup of baby kale or spinach

- ¾ cup unsweetened vanilla almond milk

- One cup of ice

Instructions

1. Add everything to a blender or high-speed food processor and blend until you get a smooth consistency. Enjoy!

CHOCOLATE BANANA DRINK

Ingredients

- Six ounces of carob-flavored soy milk (can be substituted with fortified cocoa)

- One banana, diced and frozen

- One pinch of cinnamon

Instructions

1. Combine everything in a blender and blend until smooth. Serve immediately.

KIWIFRUIT SHAKE

Ingredients

- 4 cups non-fat vanilla vegan yogurt, frozen
- 2 sliced kiwifruit

Instructions

1. Add both ingredients to a blender or food processor and blend until smooth. Serve.

LEMON QUINOA SALAD

Ingredients

- One cup of lentils, cooked
- One cup of quinoa, cooked
- Three tablespoons of olive oil
- One minced garlic clove
- Half a cup of yellow bell pepper, chopped
- Half a cup of red bell pepper, chopped
- ¼ cup freshly squeezed lemon juice
- ¼ cup red onion, chopped
- Salt to taste

Instructions

1. Combine all the ingredients (except salt) in a large bowl. Season with salt to taste.

2. You can season with more grounded pepper if you wish. Serve.

MUSHROOM & ONION GRAVY

Ingredients

- 2-3 cups of spring water
- ½ cup mushroom
- 1 tsp sea salt
- ½ cup onion
- ½ tsp oregano
- ¼ cup cayenne
- ½ tsp thyme
- 2 tbsp grapeseed oil
- 3 tbsp garbanzo bean flour
- 1 tsp onion powder

Instructions

1. Start by pouring the grapeseed oil into your frying pan. Then set it on the stove over medium or high heat.

2. Once the oil is a bit hot, add the onion and mushroom and sauté for a minute. Then add the other seasonings and spices, except the cayenne.

3. Sauté for five minutes, then add 2 cups of spring water and the cayenne. Stir well to mix and allow to boil.

4. While you're waiting, sift in the flour little by little, then use a whisk to stir it well in order to reduce lumps.

5. Continue cooking until it boils. You can add more water if you want but don't add not more than one cup. Serve.

GINGER TEA

Ingredients

- 1 pinch cayenne
- 1 thumb fresh ginger root (can be substituted with the powder)
- 4 cups spring water
- 2 tbsp fresh lime juice
- 2 sprigs of new organic dill weed
- Raw agave to taste

Instructions

1. Start by boiling the spring water.
2. While you're waiting, peel the ginger root, then chop it into tiny pieces and add to the boiling water. Also, add the weed.
3. Let it cook for 5 minutes, then strain the tea into a glass jar. Add the lime juice and cayenne and stir.
4. Finally, add the agave to taste. You can have it either hot or cold.

TASTY PANINI

Ingredients

- 1 tsp cinnamon
- ¼ cup natural peanut butter
- ¼ cup raisin
- ¼ cup hot water
- Whole grain bread, 2 slices
- 1 ripe banana, peeled and chopped
- 2 tsp cacao powder

Instructions

1. Start by pouring the hot water into a bowl. Add the cinnamon, raisin, and cacao powder and combine.
2. Next, spread the peanut butter on each of the bread slices.
3. Place the chopped banana on the toast.
4. Next, transfer the raisin mixture into a blender and blend until smooth. Spread on the sandwich. Enjoy!

BASIC POLENTA

Ingredients

- One and a half cups of coarse cornmeal
- Five cups of water
- ¾ tsp salt

Instructions

1. Start by pouring the water into a saucepan. Put it on a stove and set to low heat.
2. Gradually add the cornmeal into the water. Then stir until creamy. This might take a couple of minutes.
3. Season with the salt, then transfer the polenta into a bowl. Refrigerate for an hour, then serve.

ELECTRIC SALAD

Ingredients

- 1 cup cherry tomatoes
- 2 red onions
- 1 handful romaine lettuce
- 1 lime (you will need the juice)
- 1 cup kale, chopped
- 3 jalapenos
- Olive oil
- 1 yellow pepper
- 1 orange pepper

Instructions

1. The first thing is to wash and rinse all the ingredients if you have not already done so. Once dry, cut them into smaller pieces.
2. Combine everything in a bowl and drizzle with the lemon juice and oil. Enjoy!

QUINOA PORRIDGE

Ingredients

- ½ tsp cayenne
- ½ lime (you will need to grate the skin)
- 1 cup dry quinoa
- 2 cups water
- ½ cup coconut milk (can be substituted with cream if you wish)
- Cloves to taste
- ½ handful assorted nuts and seeds (optional)

Instructions

1. Prepare the quinoa according to the instructions on the package.

2. After that, pour it into a saucepan (this should be after you have drained the quinoa). Then add the cloves and cayenne. Stir well to combine.

3. Next, add the milk and grated lime (you can also add grated apple if you wish). Stir well to mix.

4. Top with nuts and seeds. Enjoy!

ALKALINE MILLET

Ingredients

- ½ tsp sea salt
- 2 ½ cup water
- 1 cup millet

Instructions

1. The first thing is to dry sauté the millet until golden brown. Then add in the water and salt.

2. Bring the mixture to a boil, then simmer until the water is absorbed. This usually takes about 30 minutes but it could be more depending on the heat.

3. Let everything cool with the lid on. Serve and enjoy!

ZUCCHINI AND HEART MUSHROOM SOUP

Ingredients

- 1 medium zucchini, chopped
- 1 medium-sized onion, chopped (if you eat onion a lot, then you can use a large onion instead)
- 2 bay leaves
- Any vegetable stock of your choice (ideally, homemade)
- 1 tsp grapeseed oil
- 1 lb mushroom, mixed and chopped
- Cayenne pepper to taste
- Sea salt to taste
- Sweet basil to taste

Instructions

1. Start by setting your stove to medium heat. Set a pan with a heavy base on top of the stove, then add the grapeseed oil. Once it gets a little hot, add in the onion and sauté for 5 minutes.

2. Next, add the mushrooms, basil, and bay leaves. Allow it to cook for an additional five minutes, then add the zucchini. Cook until the vegetables release their juices. This might take up to 10-15 minutes.

3. Now, pour in the vegetable stock and bring to a boil. Then reduce the heat and simmer for five minutes.

4. Finally, remove the bay leaves from the soup before seasoning with salt and pepper. Serve!

KALE SALAD & HEMP RANCH

Ingredients

- One teaspoon of dill
- Half a teaspoon of sea salt

- Half a cup of hemp seeds

- Two tablespoons of squeezed lime juice

- Half butternut squash, cubed

- Six cups of chopped kale

- Two teaspoons of salt

- One to two tablespoons of grapeseed oil

Instructions

1. Switch on the oven and heat it to up to 350-400 degrees F.

2. Put the hemp seeds, dill, and lime juice in a blender and blend until smooth. You can also use a food processor.

3. Now, toss the kale and squash in the grapeseed oil and add the sea salt. Transfer to a baking dish and roast for 15 to 20 minutes or until cooked. You will know this when the kale gets crispy.

4. Allow to cook, then you can top with dressings.

AVOCADO LETTUCE WRAPS

Ingredients

- One teaspoon of sea salt
- Two avocados, sliced
- One teaspoon of fresh lime juice
- Twelve romaine lettuce leaves
- Two diced bell peppers
- Half red onion (should be diced and sliced)
- Three plum tomatoes, chopped
- One to two teaspoons of cayenne pepper

Instructions

1. Mix all the ingredients in a bowl except the romaine lettuce.
2. Next, you want to wash the lettuce separately. Allow it to dry.
3. Now, place the dry leaves on a plate or dish in such a way that each one forms a natural scoop.

4. Next, pour the mixture you prepared from step one into each leaf so that it fills it. Now, you have your avocado lettuce wraps. Enjoy!

RYE TOMATO & AVOCADO SANDWICH

Ingredients

- Two slices of rye bread
- Two sliced plum tomatoes
- One avocado, sliced
- One to two teaspoons of sea salt
- One to three tablespoons of olive oil
- Half a cup of dandelion greens or purslane

Instructions

1. Place the avocado slices on top of the bread slices.
2. Next, drizzle with olive oil. It should go on top of the avocado.
3. Now, arrange the tomato slices on top of the avocados. You can sprinkle some salt if you wish.

4. Finally, top with purslane. Enjoy your sandwich.

SWEET POTATO & PEANUT CURRY

Ingredients

- A piece of thumb-sized ginger, grated

- 200g bag of spinach

- One tablespoon of coconut oil

- Two cloves of garlic, grated

- One onion, chopped

- One lime, juiced

- 400ml can of coconut milk

- Three tablespoons of Thai red curry paste (ensure it's vegan, you can check for this on the label or packaging)

- One tablespoon of peanut butter

- 500g of sweet potato (after peeling, cut it into small chunks)

- Water

Instructions

1. Start by melting the coconut oil in a saucepan over medium heat. Then add the onion and saute for 4-5 minutes.
2. Next, add in the garlic cloves and ginger and cook for another one minute until the fragrance is released.
3. Now, stir in the other ingredients - curry paste, peanut butter, coconut milk, and sweet potato. Add in about 200 ml of water.
4. Allow the mixture to boil, then reduce the heat and simmer for an additional 20 minutes or until the potatoes become soft. The cover of the saucepan should be removed during this period.
5. Finally, stir in the spinach and lime juice and add your favorite seasoning. Serve alone or with cooked rice (ideally, brown rice or whole grain rice)

MANGO & AVOCADO SALSA

Ingredients

- One garlic clove, minced
- Two tablespoons of fresh lime juice
- One ripe mango (make sure to peel and dice it before use)
- One jalapeno, seeded and diced
- One plum tomato, diced
- One medium Hass avocado, diced
- Half a tablespoon of olive oil
- Two tablespoons of fresh lime juice
- ¼ cup fresh cilantro, chopped
- ¼ cup red onion, chopped
- Pepper and kosher salt to taste

Instructions

1. Mix all the ingredients together in a bowl. Then put
   it in a refrigerator to marinate for about 30 minutes.
   Enjoy.

ZUCCHINI & PLUM TOMATOES

Ingredients

- Half a tablespoon of Herbes de Provence (you can
  find how to make this online)
- One medium-sized zucchini (cut into bits)
- Five medium-sized fresh plum tomatoes, diced
- Two tablespoons of extra virgin olive oil
- Five garlic cloves, smashed
- Fresh pepper and kosher salt to taste

Instructions

1. Pour the olive oil into a large non-stick skillet and
    heat. Set the stove to medium-high heat.

2. Add in the garlic and sauté until it turns golden. This
    should take about a minute or two.

3. Now, add in salt and pepper followed by zucchini.

4. Leave it to cook for 4 to 5 minutes on each side.
    Then introduce the plum tomatoes and Herbes de
    Provence. You can add additional salt if you desire.

5. Reduce the heat and simmer for 5 to 10 minutes.
    Serve.

BAKED BANANAS

Ingredients

- 1 banana (ideally, it should be medium ripped; cut it
  into half lengthwise)
- Half a tablespoon of honey
- Cinnamon to taste

Instructions

1. Start by preheating the oven to 400 degrees F.

2. Arrange the banana halves on a foil or oven-safe dish. Sprinkle with honey and cinnamon.

3. Cover tight with foil, then place it in the oven and allow to bake for 10-15 minutes. Enjoy!

4. Optionally, you can serve with light ice cream or whipped cream.

BUTTERNUT SQUASH LENTIL SOUP

Ingredients

- One bay leaf
- One large onion, diced
- One celery stalk, diced

- One medium-sized carrot, diced
- Half a tablespoon of olive oil
- Six cups of vegetable broth
- Two leeks (we will need only the white part; clean and chop into smaller pieces)
- Two tablespoons of tomato paste
- One pound of butternut, peeled and diced into half inches
- Two ounces of green lentils (this is equivalent to ⅓ cup)
- Three cups of packed chopped lacinato kale (the stems should be removed)
- Half a teaspoon of kosher salt

Instructions

1. Start by heating a Dutch oven or some other heavy pot over medium heat.
2. Once it gets hot, add the olive oil, and follow up with the onions, celery, leeks, and carrots. Reduce the heat and let it cook for 4-5 minutes as you stir it.

3. Now, add in the tomato paste and let it cook for an additional two minutes while stirring.

4. Pour in the vegetable broth, lentils, and bay leaf and allow to boil. Then reduce the heat, cover the pot and simmer for about 20 minutes.

5. Introduce the butternut and cook until tender. This should take up to 15 minutes or more.

6. Remove the bay leaf, then add salt and pepper as seasoning. Now, add in the kale and allow to cook for 5 to 7 minutes or until the kale becomes tender.

Conclusion

We will draw the curtains here. Like I said earlier, a proper Lyme diet should boost your immune system, fight off inflammation, detox your organs, and regulate your hormones. The Dr Barbara diet ticks all the boxes.

In addition to the above benefits, following the Dr Barbara Alkaline Diet can help reduce joint pain and swelling, ease headaches, improve memory and concentration, promote thyroid and adrenal function, replace bad gut bacteria with the good ones, and improve your energy level.

Finally, you should consider a plant-based way of eating a lifestyle rather than a diet. This will make it easier to make a switch and not be disappointed when you don't see results immediately.

www.ingramcontent.com/pod-product-compliance
Lightning Source LLC
Chambersburg PA
CBHW051655250726
48653CB00007B/2675